I0425313

My Grilling Recipes
by

_____

Notes & Pictures

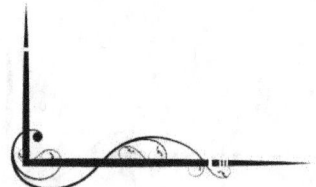

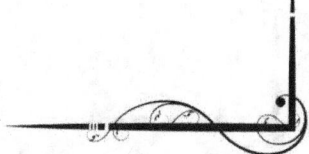

Prep Time _____

Cook Time _____

Recipe _____

Ingredients:

_____   _____

_____   _____

_____   _____

_____   _____

_____   _____

_____   _____

Directions:

_____

_____

_____

_____

_____

_____

_____

_____

Notes:

Recipe_____

Prep Time _____
Cook Time _____

Ingredients:

_____   _____
_____   _____
_____   _____
_____   _____
_____   _____

Directions:

_____
_____
_____
_____
_____
_____
_____
_____
_____

Notes:

Prep Time _____

Cook Time _____

Recipe_____

Ingredients:

_____ _____

_____ _____

_____ _____

_____ _____

_____ _____

Directions:

_____

_____

_____

_____

_____

_____

_____

_____

_____

Notes:

Recipe_____

Ingredients:

_____ _____

_____ _____

_____ _____

_____ _____

_____ _____

Directions:

_____

_____

_____

_____

_____

_____

_____

_____

Notes:

Recipe _____

Ingredients:

_____ _____

_____ _____

_____ _____

_____ _____

_____ _____

Directions:

_____

_____

_____

_____

_____

_____

_____

_____

Notes:

Recipe_____

Prep Time _____
Cook Time _____

Ingredients:

_____ _____

_____ _____

_____ _____

_____ _____

_____ _____

Directions:

_____

_____

_____

_____

_____

_____

_____

_____

Notes:

Prep Time _____

Cook Time _____

Recipe_____

Ingredients:

_____   _____

_____   _____

_____   _____

_____   _____

_____   _____

                    _____

Directions:

_____

_____

_____

_____

_____

_____

_____

_____

_____

Notes:

Prep Time _____

Cook Time _____

Recipe _____

Ingredients:

_____   _____

_____   _____

_____   _____

_____   _____

_____   _____

Directions:

_____

_____

_____

_____

_____

_____

_____

_____

Notes:

Prep Time _____

Cook Time _____

Recipe_____

Ingredients:

_____   _____

_____   _____

_____   _____

_____   _____

_____   _____

Directions:

_____

_____

_____

_____

_____

_____

_____

_____

Notes:

Recipe_____

Ingredients:

_____ _____
_____ _____
_____ _____
_____ _____
_____ _____
_____ _____

Directions:

_____
_____
_____
_____
_____
_____
_____
_____

Notes:

Prep Time _____

Cook Time _____

Recipe_____

Ingredients:

_____   _____

_____   _____

_____   _____

_____   _____

_____   _____

_____

Directions:

_____

_____

_____

_____

_____

_____

_____

_____

Notes:

Recipe _____

Prep Time _____

Cook Time _____

Ingredients:

_____ _____

_____ _____

_____ _____

_____ _____

_____ _____

Directions:

_____

_____

_____

_____

_____

_____

_____

_____

_____

Notes:

Prep Time _____

Cook Time _____

Recipe_____

Ingredients:

_____ _____

_____ _____

_____ _____

_____ _____

_____ _____

_____ _____

Directions:

_____

_____

_____

_____

_____

_____

_____

_____

Notes:

Prep Time _____

Cook Time _____

Recipe_____

Ingredients:

_____   _____

_____   _____

_____   _____

_____   _____

_____   _____

Directions:

_____

_____

_____

_____

_____

_____

_____

Notes:

Recipe_____

Ingredients:

_____   _____

_____   _____

_____   _____

_____   _____

_____   _____

Directions:

_____

_____

_____

_____

_____

_____

_____

_____

Notes:

Prep Time _____

Cook Time _____

Recipe_____

Ingredients:

_____   _____

_____   _____

_____   _____

_____   _____

_____   _____

_____   _____

Directions:

_____

_____

_____

_____

_____

_____

_____

_____

_____

Notes:

Recipe_____

Ingredients:

_____   _____
_____   _____
_____   _____
_____   _____
_____   _____
_____   _____

Directions:

_____
_____
_____
_____
_____
_____
_____
_____
_____

Notes:

Recipe_____

Ingredients:

_____   _____

_____   _____

_____   _____

_____   _____

_____   _____

_____   _____

Directions:

_____

_____

_____

_____

_____

_____

_____

Notes:

Prep Time _____

Cook Time _____

Recipe_____

Ingredients:

_____ _____

_____ _____

_____ _____

_____ _____

_____ _____

Directions:

_____

_____

_____

_____

_____

_____

_____

_____

Notes:

Recipe_____

Ingredients:

_____   _____

_____   _____

_____   _____

_____   _____

_____   _____

_____   _____

Directions:

_____

_____

_____

_____

_____

_____

_____

_____

Notes:

Prep Time _____

Cook Time _____

Recipe_____

Ingredients:

_____   _____

_____   _____

_____   _____

_____   _____

_____   _____

_____   _____

Directions:

_____

_____

_____

_____

_____

_____

_____

_____

_____

Notes:

Recipe_____

Prep Time _____
Cook Time _____

Ingredients:

_____ _____
_____ _____
_____ _____
_____ _____
_____ _____
_____ _____

Directions:

_____
_____
_____
_____
_____
_____
_____
_____
_____

Notes:

Recipe _____

Ingredients:

_____ _____

_____ _____

_____ _____

_____ _____

_____ _____

_____ _____

Directions:

_____

_____

_____

_____

_____

_____

_____

_____

Notes:

Prep Time _____

Cook Time _____

Recipe_____

Ingredients:

_____ _____

_____ _____

_____ _____

_____ _____

_____ _____

_____

Directions:

_____

_____

_____

_____

_____

_____

_____

_____

_____

Notes:

Recipe_____

Prep Time _____
Cook Time _____

Ingredients:

_____ _____

_____ _____

_____ _____

_____ _____

_____ _____

_____

Directions:

_____

_____

_____

_____

_____

_____

_____

_____

_____

Notes:

Prep Time _____

Cook Time _____

Recipe_____

Ingredients:

_____   _____

_____   _____

_____   _____

_____   _____

_____   _____

_____

Directions:

_____

_____

_____

_____

_____

_____

_____

_____

_____

Notes:

Recipe_____

Ingredients:

_____ _____

_____ _____

_____ _____

_____ _____

_____ _____

Directions:

_____

_____

_____

_____

_____

_____

_____

_____

Notes:

Recipe_____

Prep Time _____

Cook Time _____

Ingredients:

_____   _____

_____   _____

_____   _____

_____   _____

_____   _____

Directions:

_____

_____

_____

_____

_____

_____

_____

_____

_____

Notes:

Prep Time _____
Cook Time _____

Recipe _____

Ingredients:

_____ _____
_____ _____
_____ _____
_____ _____
_____ _____

Directions:

_____
_____
_____
_____
_____
_____
_____
_____

Notes:

Prep Time _____

Cook Time _____

Recipe_____

Ingredients:

_____   _____

_____   _____

_____   _____

_____   _____

_____   _____

_____   _____

Directions:

_____

_____

_____

_____

_____

_____

_____

_____

_____

Notes:

Prep Time _____

Cook Time _____

Recipe _____

Ingredients:

_____   _____

_____   _____

_____   _____

_____   _____

_____   _____

Directions:

_____

_____

_____

_____

_____

_____

_____

_____

Notes:

Prep Time _____

Cook Time _____

Recipe_____

Ingredients:

_____ _____

_____ _____

_____ _____

_____ _____

_____ _____

Directions:

_____

_____

_____

_____

_____

_____

_____

_____

Notes:

Recipe_____

Ingredients:

_____ _____

_____ _____

_____ _____

_____ _____

_____ _____

_____ _____

Directions:

_____

_____

_____

_____

_____

_____

_____

_____

_____

Notes:

Prep Time _____

Cook Time _____

Recipe_____

Ingredients:

_____   _____

_____   _____

_____   _____

_____   _____

_____   _____

Directions:

_____

_____

_____

_____

_____

_____

_____

Notes:

Prep Time _____

Cook Time _____

Recipe_____

Ingredients:

_____ _____

_____ _____

_____ _____

_____ _____

_____ _____

_____

Directions:

_____

_____

_____

_____

_____

_____

_____

_____

_____

Notes:

Prep Time _____

Cook Time _____

Recipe _____

Ingredients:

_____   _____

_____   _____

_____   _____

_____   _____

_____   _____

Directions:

_____

_____

_____

_____

_____

_____

_____

_____

Notes:

Prep Time _____

Cook Time _____

Recipe_____

Ingredients:

_____   _____

_____   _____

_____   _____

_____   _____

_____   _____

_____

Directions:

_____

_____

_____

_____

_____

_____

_____

_____

Notes:

Recipe_____

Ingredients:

_____   _____

_____   _____

_____   _____

_____   _____

_____   _____

_____   _____

Directions:

_____

_____

_____

_____

_____

_____

_____

_____

_____

Notes:

Prep Time _____

Cook Time _____

Recipe _____

Ingredients:

_____ _____

_____ _____

_____ _____

_____ _____

_____ _____

_____ _____

Directions:

_____

_____

_____

_____

_____

_____

_____

_____

_____

Notes:

Recipe_____

Ingredients:

_____   _____

_____   _____

_____   _____

_____   _____

_____   _____

Directions:

_____

_____

_____

_____

_____

_____

_____

_____

Notes:

Prep Time _____

Cook Time _____

Recipe_____

Ingredients:

_____   _____

_____   _____

_____   _____

_____   _____

_____   _____

Directions:

_____

_____

_____

_____

_____

_____

_____

_____

Notes:

Prep Time _____

Cook Time _____

Recipe _____

Ingredients:

_____ _____

_____ _____

_____ _____

_____ _____

_____ _____

_____ _____

Directions:

_____

_____

_____

_____

_____

_____

_____

_____

Notes:

Recipe_____

Prep Time _____
Cook Time _____

Ingredients:

_____ _____

_____ _____

_____ _____

_____ _____

_____ _____

_____ _____

Directions:

_____

_____

_____

_____

_____

_____

_____

_____

_____

Notes:

Prep Time _____

Cook Time _____

Recipe_____

Ingredients:

_____ _____

_____ _____

_____ _____

_____ _____

_____ _____

Directions:

_____

_____

_____

_____

_____

_____

_____

_____

Notes:

Prep Time _____

Cook Time _____

Recipe_____

Ingredients:

_____   _____

_____   _____

_____   _____

_____   _____

_____   _____

_____   _____

Directions:

_____

_____

_____

_____

_____

_____

_____

_____

_____

Notes:

Recipe_____

Ingredients:

_____   _____
_____   _____
_____   _____
_____   _____
_____   _____

Directions:

_____
_____
_____
_____
_____
_____
_____

Notes:

Prep Time _____

Cook Time _____

Recipe _____

Ingredients:

_____ _____

_____ _____

_____ _____

_____ _____

_____ _____

_____

Directions:

_____

_____

_____

_____

_____

_____

_____

_____

_____

Notes:

Recipe_____

Ingredients:

_____   _____
_____   _____
_____   _____
_____   _____
_____   _____

Directions:

_____
_____
_____
_____
_____
_____
_____
_____
_____

Notes:

Prep Time _____

Cook Time _____

Recipe_____

Ingredients:

_____   _____

_____   _____

_____   _____

_____   _____

_____   _____

_____   _____

Directions:

_____

_____

_____

_____

_____

_____

_____

_____

_____

Notes:

Prep Time _____

Cook Time _____

Recipe_____

Ingredients:

_____ _____

_____ _____

_____ _____

_____ _____

_____ _____

_____ _____

Directions:

_____

_____

_____

_____

_____

_____

_____

_____

_____

Notes:

Recipe_____

Ingredients:

_____ _____

_____ _____

_____ _____

_____ _____

_____ _____

_____ _____

Directions:

_____

_____

_____

_____

_____

_____

_____

_____

_____

Notes:

Prep Time _____

Cook Time _____

Recipe_____

Ingredients:

_____ _____

_____ _____

_____ _____

_____ _____

_____ _____

Directions:

_____

_____

_____

_____

_____

_____

_____

_____

Notes:

Prep Time _____

Cook Time _____

Recipe_____

Ingredients:

_____   _____

_____   _____

_____   _____

_____   _____

_____   _____

                                _____

Directions:

_____

_____

_____

_____

_____

_____

_____

_____

_____

Notes:

Recipe_____

Ingredients:

_____ _____

_____ _____

_____ _____

_____ _____

_____ _____

_____ _____

Directions:

_____

_____

_____

_____

_____

_____

_____

_____

_____

Notes:

Prep Time _____

Cook Time _____

Recipe_____

Ingredients:

_____   _____

_____   _____

_____   _____

_____   _____

_____   _____

_____

Directions:

_____

_____

_____

_____

_____

_____

_____

_____

_____

Notes:

Recipe_____

Ingredients:

_____   _____

_____   _____

_____   _____

_____   _____

_____   _____

_____   _____

Directions:

_____

_____

_____

_____

_____

_____

_____

_____

_____

Notes:

Prep Time _____

Cook Time _____

Recipe_____

Ingredients:

_____   _____

_____   _____

_____   _____

_____   _____

_____   _____

_____   _____

Directions:

_____

_____

_____

_____

_____

_____

_____

_____

_____

Notes:

Recipe_____

Prep Time _____
Cook Time _____

Ingredients:

_____ _____
_____ _____
_____ _____
_____ _____
_____ _____
_____ _____

Directions:

_____
_____
_____
_____
_____
_____
_____
_____
_____

Notes:

Prep Time _____
Cook Time _____

Recipe_____

Ingredients:

_____   _____
_____   _____
_____   _____
_____   _____
_____   _____

Directions:

_____
_____
_____
_____
_____
_____
_____
_____

Notes:

Prep Time _____

Cook Time _____

Recipe_____

Ingredients:

_____ _____

_____ _____

_____ _____

_____ _____

_____ _____

Directions:

_____

_____

_____

_____

_____

_____

_____

_____

Notes:

Recipe_____

Ingredients:

_____   _____

_____   _____

_____   _____

_____   _____

_____   _____

_____   _____

Directions:

_____

_____

_____

_____

_____

_____

_____

_____

_____

Notes:

Prep Time _____
Cook Time _____

Recipe _____

Ingredients:

_____ _____

_____ _____

_____ _____

_____ _____

_____ _____

_____ _____

Directions:

_____

_____

_____

_____

_____

_____

_____

_____

_____

Notes:

Prep Time _____

Cook Time _____

Recipe_____

Ingredients:

_____ _____

_____ _____

_____ _____

_____ _____

_____ _____

_____ _____

Directions:

_____

_____

_____

_____

_____

_____

_____

_____

_____

Notes:

Prep Time _____

Cook Time _____

Recipe_____

Ingredients:

_____   _____

_____   _____

_____   _____

_____   _____

_____   _____

Directions:

_____

_____

_____

_____

_____

_____

_____

_____

Notes:

Prep Time _____

Cook Time _____

Recipe_____

Ingredients:

_____   _____

_____   _____

_____   _____

_____   _____

_____   _____

_____   _____

Directions:

_____

_____

_____

_____

_____

_____

_____

_____

Notes:

Recipe_____

Prep Time _____
Cook Time _____

Ingredients:

_____ _____
_____ _____
_____ _____
_____ _____
_____ _____
_____ _____

Directions:

_____
_____
_____
_____
_____
_____
_____
_____
_____

Notes:

Recipe_____

Ingredients:

_____   _____

_____   _____

_____   _____

_____   _____

_____   _____

   _____

Directions:

_____

_____

_____

_____

_____

_____

_____

_____

_____

Notes:

Recipe

Prep Time _____

Cook Time _____

Ingredients:

_____ _____

_____ _____

_____ _____

_____ _____

_____ _____

Directions:

_____

_____

_____

_____

_____

_____

_____

_____

Notes:

Recipe_____

Prep Time _____
Cook Time _____

Ingredients:

_____ _____

_____ _____

_____ _____

_____ _____

_____ _____

_____

Directions:

_____

_____

_____

_____

_____

_____

_____

_____

Notes:

Recipe_____

Ingredients:

_____   _____

_____   _____

_____   _____

_____   _____

_____   _____

_____   _____

Directions:

_____

_____

_____

_____

_____

_____

_____

_____

_____

Notes:

Recipe_____

Ingredients:

_____ _____

_____ _____

_____ _____

_____ _____

_____ _____

_____

Directions:

_____

_____

_____

_____

_____

_____

_____

_____

_____

Notes:

Prep Time _____

Cook Time _____

Recipe_____

Ingredients:

_____   _____

_____   _____

_____   _____

_____   _____

_____   _____

Directions:

_____

_____

_____

_____

_____

_____

_____

_____

_____

Notes:

Prep Time _____

Cook Time _____

Recipe _____

Ingredients:

_____   _____

_____   _____

_____   _____

_____   _____

_____   _____

_____

Directions:

_____

_____

_____

_____

_____

_____

_____

_____

_____

Notes:

Prep Time _____

Cook Time _____

Recipe_____

Ingredients:

_____   _____

_____   _____

_____   _____

_____   _____

_____   _____

_____   _____

Directions:

_____

_____

_____

_____

_____

_____

_____

_____

_____

Notes:

Recipe_____

Cook Time _____

Ingredients:

_____   _____

_____   _____

_____   _____

_____   _____

_____   _____

_____   _____

Directions:

_____

_____

_____

_____

_____

_____

_____

_____

_____

Notes:

Recipe _____

Ingredients:

_____   _____

_____   _____

_____   _____

_____   _____

_____   _____

_____   _____

Directions:

_____

_____

_____

_____

_____

_____

_____

_____

_____

Notes:

Prep Time _____

Cook Time _____

Recipe _____

Ingredients:

_____   _____

_____   _____

_____   _____

_____   _____

_____   _____

_____   _____

Directions:

_____

_____

_____

_____

_____

_____

_____

_____

_____

Notes:

Prep Time _____

Cook Time _____

Recipe _____

Ingredients:

_____ _____

_____ _____

_____ _____

_____ _____

_____ _____

Directions:

_____

_____

_____

_____

_____

_____

_____

_____

Notes:

Recipe_____

Ingredients:

_____   _____
_____   _____
_____   _____
_____   _____
_____   _____
_____

Directions:

_____
_____
_____
_____
_____
_____
_____
_____
_____

Notes:

Recipe_____

Prep Time _____
Cook Time _____

Ingredients:

_____ _____

_____ _____

_____ _____

_____ _____

_____ _____

Directions:

_____

_____

_____

_____

_____

_____

_____

_____

Notes:

Prep Time _____

Cook Time _____

Recipe_____

Ingredients:

_____ _____

_____ _____

_____ _____

_____ _____

_____ _____

_____

Directions:

_____

_____

_____

_____

_____

_____

_____

_____

_____

Notes:

Prep Time _____

Cook Time _____

Recipe_____

Ingredients:

_____   _____

_____   _____

_____   _____

_____   _____

_____   _____

Directions:

_____

_____

_____

_____

_____

_____

_____

_____

Notes:

Recipe_____

Ingredients:

_____ _____
_____ _____
_____ _____
_____ _____
_____ _____
_____ _____

Directions:

_____
_____
_____
_____
_____
_____
_____
_____
_____

Notes:

Prep Time _____

Cook Time _____

Recipe_____

Ingredients:

_____   _____

_____   _____

_____   _____

_____   _____

_____   _____

_____   _____

Directions:

_____

_____

_____

_____

_____

_____

_____

_____

_____

Notes:

Prep Time _____

Cook Time _____

Recipe_____

Ingredients:

_____ _____

_____ _____

_____ _____

_____ _____

_____ _____

Directions:

_____

_____

_____

_____

_____

_____

_____

_____

Notes:

Recipe_____

Ingredients:

_____   _____

_____   _____

_____   _____

_____   _____

_____   _____

_____   _____

Directions:

_____

_____

_____

_____

_____

_____

_____

_____

_____

Notes:

Prep Time _____

Cook Time _____

Recipe_____

Ingredients:

_____   _____

_____   _____

_____   _____

_____   _____

_____   _____

_____   _____

Directions:

_____

_____

_____

_____

_____

_____

_____

_____

_____

Notes:

Recipe_____

Ingredients:

_____   _____

_____   _____

_____   _____

_____   _____

_____   _____

Directions:

_____

_____

_____

_____

_____

_____

_____

_____

_____

Notes:

Prep Time _____
Cook Time _____

Recipe_____

Ingredients:

_____ _____

_____ _____

_____ _____

_____ _____

_____ _____

Directions:

_____

_____

_____

_____

_____

_____

_____

_____

Notes:

Recipe_____

Ingredients:

_____   _____
_____   _____
_____   _____
_____   _____
_____   _____
_____

Directions:

_____
_____
_____
_____
_____
_____
_____
_____

Notes:

Prep Time _____

Cook Time _____

Recipe_____

Ingredients:

_____ _____

_____ _____

_____ _____

_____ _____

_____ _____

Directions:

_____

_____

_____

_____

_____

_____

_____

_____

Notes:

Recipe_____

Prep Time _____
Cook Time _____

Ingredients:

_____   _____
_____   _____
_____   _____
_____   _____
_____   _____

Directions:

_____
_____
_____
_____
_____
_____
_____
_____
_____

Notes:

Recipe_____

Prep Time _____
Cook Time _____

Ingredients:

_____   _____

_____   _____

_____   _____

_____   _____

_____   _____

_____

Directions:

_____

_____

_____

_____

_____

_____

_____

_____

Notes:

Prep Time _____

Cook Time _____

Recipe_____

Ingredients:

_____ _____

_____ _____

_____ _____

_____ _____

_____ _____

_____ _____

Directions:

_____

_____

_____

_____

_____

_____

_____

_____

Notes:

Recipe_____

Prep Time _____
Cook Time _____

Ingredients:

_____ _____

_____ _____

_____ _____

_____ _____

_____ _____

_____ _____

Directions:

_____

_____

_____

_____

_____

_____

_____

_____

Notes:

Prep Time _____

Cook Time _____

Recipe _____

Ingredients:

_____ _____

_____ _____

_____ _____

_____ _____

_____ _____

Directions:

_____

_____

_____

_____

_____

_____

_____

_____

_____

Notes:

Prep Time _____

Cook Time _____

Recipe_____

Ingredients:

_____   _____

_____   _____

_____   _____

_____   _____

_____   _____

_____   _____

Directions:

_____

_____

_____

_____

_____

_____

_____

_____

_____

Notes:

Recipe_____

Prep Time _____
Cook Time _____

Ingredients:

_____   _____

_____   _____

_____   _____

_____   _____

_____   _____

_____   _____

Directions:

_____

_____

_____

_____

_____

_____

_____

_____

Notes:

Prep Time _____

Cook Time _____

Recipe_____

Ingredients:

_____   _____

_____   _____

_____   _____

_____   _____

_____   _____

_____   _____

Directions:

_____

_____

_____

_____

_____

_____

_____

_____

Notes:

Recipe_____

Ingredients:

_____ _____

_____ _____

_____ _____

_____ _____

_____ _____

Directions:

_____

_____

_____

_____

_____

_____

_____

Notes:

Notes & Pictures

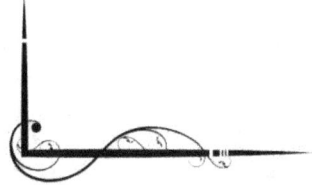

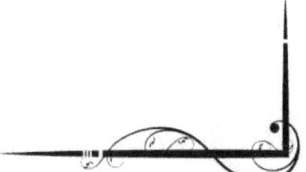

Notes & Pictures

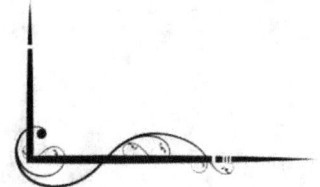

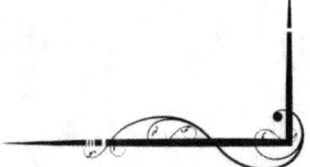

Notes & Pictures

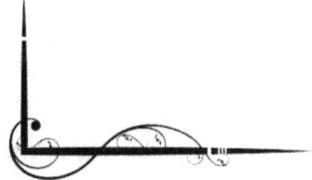
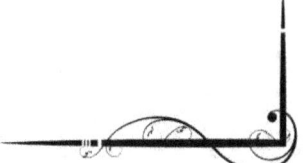

Notes & Pictures

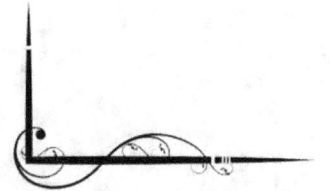

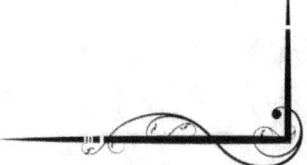

Notes & Pictures

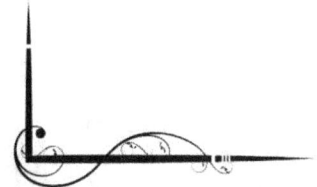
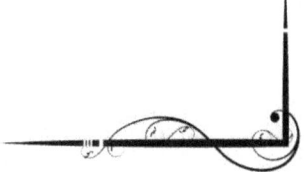

Notes & Pictures

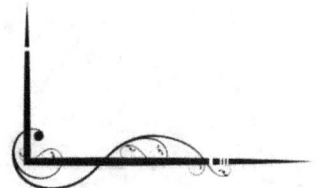
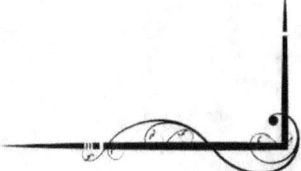

Notes & Pictures

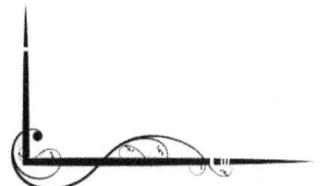
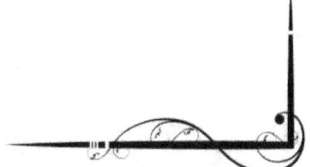

Notes & Pictures

Notes & Pictures

Notes & Pictures

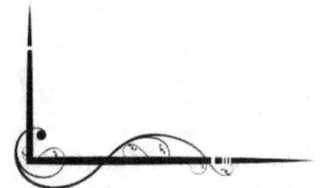

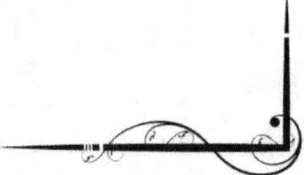

Notes & Pictures

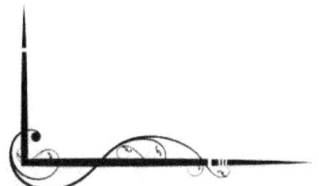
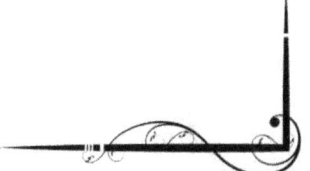

Notes & Pictures

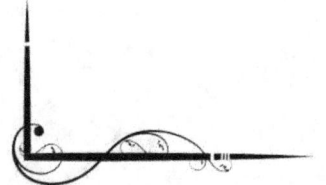

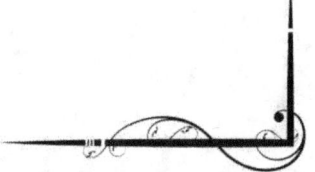

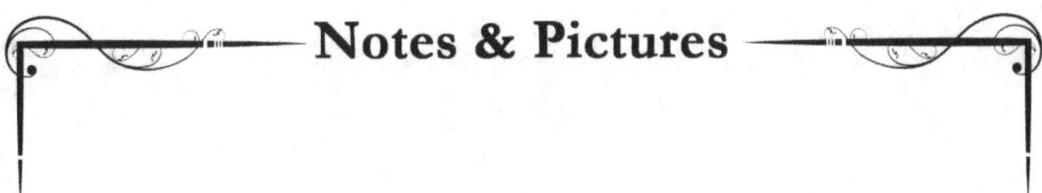

Notes & Pictures

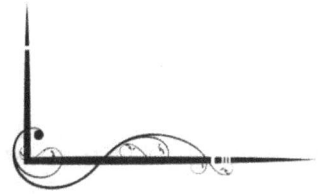
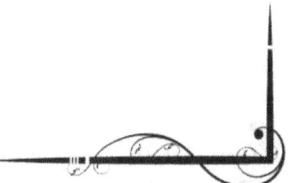

Notes & Pictures

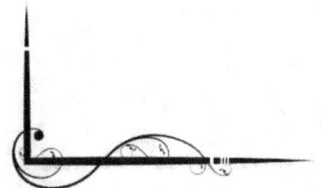

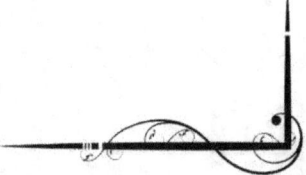

Notes & Pictures

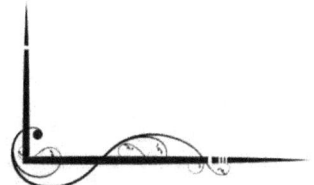

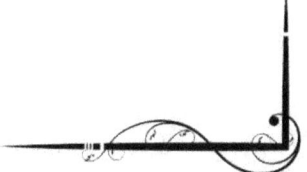

Notes & Pictures

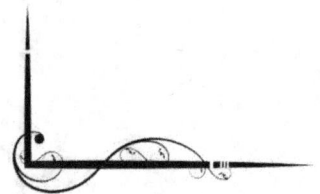

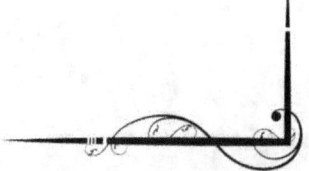

Notes & Pictures

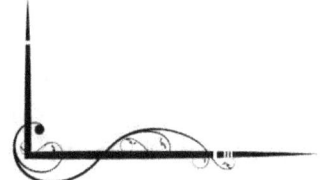
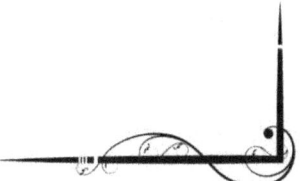

Notes & Pictures